## Copyr

© 2021 Mathias Method – All Rights Rese

No portion of this work may be reproduced or transmitted in any form or by any means, electronic or mechanical, including photocopying and recording, or by any information storage or retrieval system, without permission in writing from the author Ryan J. Mathias.

## Disclaimer

The information presented is meant to help guide participants through practices that can help individuals become stronger and healthier through proper use. This information, however, does not promise any benefits when misused or misinterpreted. Please follow the guidelines as directed.

When participating in any exercise or training program there is a possibility of physical injury. If you engage in any movements, exercises or training programs, you agree to do so at your own risk. By voluntarily participating in these activities, you assume all risk of injury to yourself and agree to release and discharge Mathias Method, Ryan J. Mathias and all other affiliates of any responsibility if injury occurs.

In addition, by following any of the suggested guidelines, protocols, templates, activities or any other information or advice given, you do so at your own risk. Do not begin any nutrition, health, exercise or training program without consulting with a Board Certified Medical Doctor and/or Registered Dietician first.

Always use spotters and any necessary safety equipment when training. It is your duty to inspect all training and safety equipment prior to each use.

By utilizing this information presented you are stating that you agree to our Terms of Use which can be read in full on MathiasMethod.com/terms-use/.

## About The Author

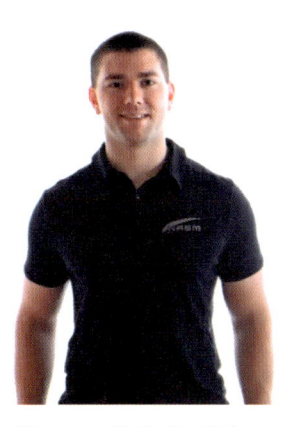

**Ryan J. Mathias**

Hi,

I'm Ryan Mathias, creator of the Mathias Method Strength System and for years I have been helping people all over the world, from total beginners to elite athletes, learn how to get stronger, perform better, and achieve their goals.

As an athlete, Strength Coach and competitive Powerlifter with 10+ years of experience, all backed by a Degree in Exercise Science, I have taken my experience and combined it with my education to bring you the best and most effective knowledge available.

I share everything I know in my books and it is my goal to help as many people as I can learn how to achieve their goals. Because I measure my success not by how many books I sell, but by how many people I help.

So, if you want to learn how to get bigger, stronger, faster, and overall perform better, then I'm your guy!

Plus, if you ever have any questions, you can email me anytime and I will do my best to help you reach your goals!

**Email:** ryan@mathiasmethod.com

I would love to hear from you!

**Join me on Social Media:** @RyanJMathias

# Books By Ryan J. Mathias

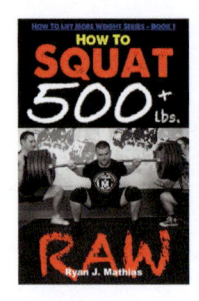

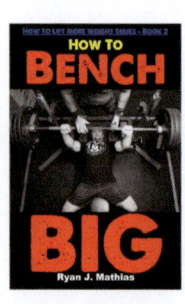

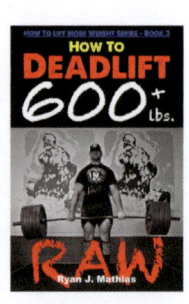

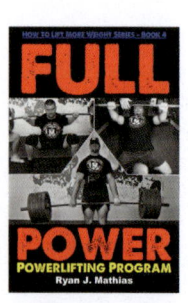

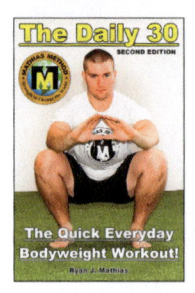

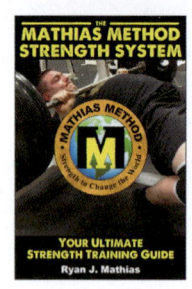

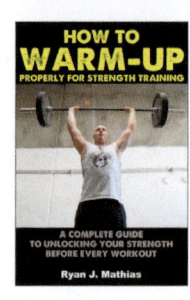

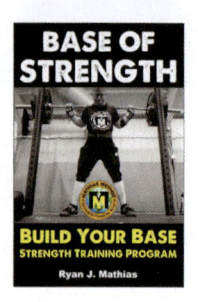

Available on

## Amazon.com

and

## StrengthWorld.store

# Table Of Contents

A Note From The Author ........................................................... 7

Developing A Base .................................................................... 9

## BASE OF STRENGTH PROGRAM — 11

Program Details ........................................................................ 13
    The Warm-Up ................................................................... 13
    Technique Work ................................................................ 14
    Main Lifts ........................................................................... 14
    Main Accessory ................................................................. 15
    Accessory Work ................................................................ 15
    Cardio/Conditioning ......................................................... 16
    Mobility Work ................................................................... 17

Weekly Training Schedule ....................................................... 19

Workouts ................................................................................. 22
    Workout 1 - Squat Training ............................................. 23
    Workout 2 - Bench Press Training .................................. 24
    Workout 3 - Deadlift Training .......................................... 25
    Workout 4 - Military Press Training ............................... 26

Program FAQ's ........................................................................ 27

Final Note ................................................................................ 31

# A Note From The Author

Strength is the base for all other Training Goals. I wish I would have known that, long ago, when I started my very own Strength Journey.

As a short, husky kid growing up with 3 brothers, I always wanted to look better and get stronger. I started off doing some PTs my dad had my brothers and I do when we were little, then eventually grew into doing some weight training.

All along the way, I didn't have much guidance on how to properly approach my goals. I would stop eating fat entirely as a young teen to try to lose body fat and would do a tremendous amount of push-ups along with other various exercise, but I was doing it all wrong.

Even when lifting weights I was not properly shown how to lift or create a successful program. If only I would have been given a system to follow or a general plan to build upon I would have been set up for much greater success.

So, in my efforts to grow stronger, as a teen I started making my own programs. Though they were nothing like what I should have been doing.

As I learned more from my own experiences and research I would continually redevelop my program to become better and better. I would read something new to try from the internet or a magazine, then go see if it worked for me.

Many times it was a high level bodybuilding routine I would try that I was not ready for, and broke me down more than it helped me get stronger.

So, through all the struggles and failed attempts to make progress, I learned many important lessons that helped me develop an incredible base of knowledge in which to build upon.

After many years of slowly progressing I continued to develop my training programs, obtained my NASM (National Academy of Sports Medicine) Personal Training Certificate, and worked hard to get my B.S. Degree in Exercise Science, that combined helped me develop the Mathias Method Strength System.

Overall, I had a long journey to get to where I am today, but I am glad

I was able to suffer through, because I came out the other side so much stronger.

Now I am dedicated to using that knowledge to help you learn how to get stronger the right way, without the need of years worth of trial and error. Let's go get stronger!

Strength To You,

**Ryan J. Mathias**

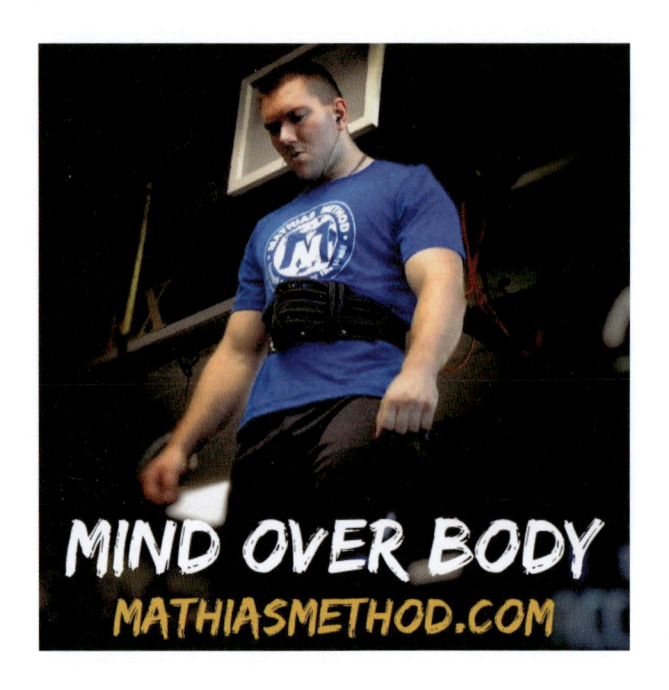

# **DEVELOPING A BASE**

As I said before, strength is the base for all other Training Goals. By becoming stronger you are better able to build muscle, lose weight, improve athleticism, prevent injury, and live a healthier lifestyle.

To accomplish anything we all need a strong base of strength. Whether you are looking to build muscle, get leaner, increase your athletic performance, or anything that involves movement, it is all the same.

Accomplishments don't occur in just one moment. They all take time and dedication, built upon a strong base. It's time to build/rebuild yours!

This is a strength based program designed to help you build a strong base of strength you can develop upon. Even if you already have built up some strength, this program can be used by individuals at any experience level, to strengthen their training foundation.

This program is meant to help anyone, get back to the basics of strength training, leading them into a stronger future!

5x5 programs are the most basic strength programs you can utilize, and they are highly effective! It's because of their simplicity and effectiveness that it is one of the most popular programs for anyone to get stronger with. There is not too much intensity, volume or complexity, making it optimal for beginners, as well as anyone else that needs to be reminded the importance of strength.

So let's get started…

# Base Of Strength Program

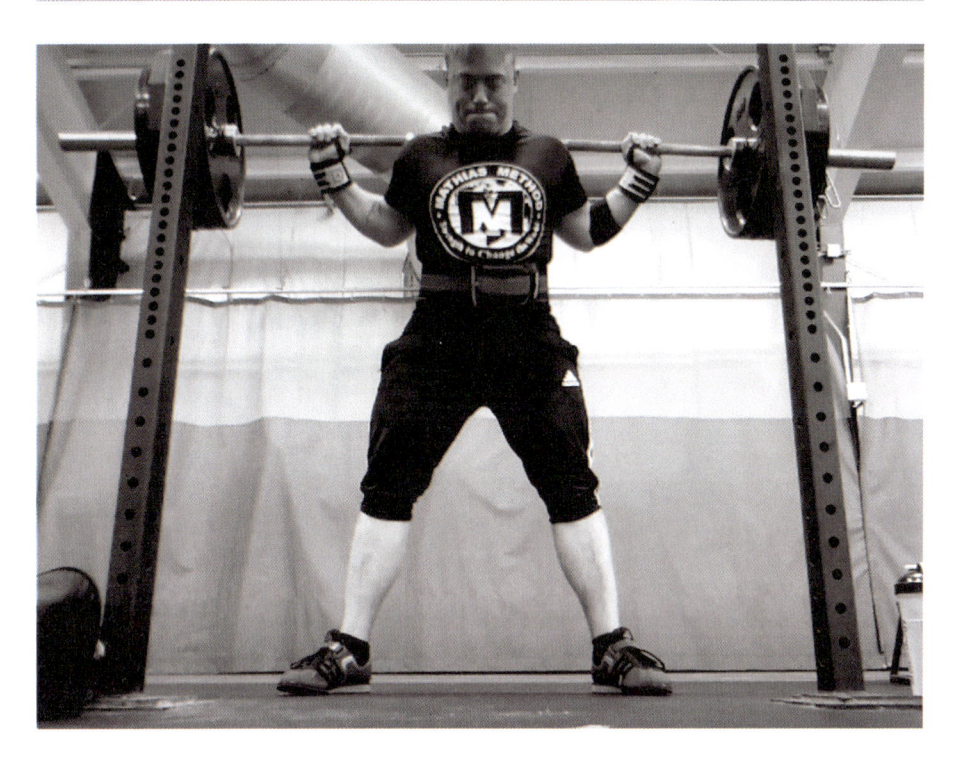

**Build Muscle and Strength
that will last for years!**

## About This Program

Base Of Strength is a simple, no non-sense approach to continuously building strength week-after-week, year-after-year! It is the perfect workout program for beginners and even advanced lifters looking to build (or re-build) a strong base.

If you want to build some serious muscle and strength that will last for years to come, this is the program you want!

With this strength training program, you will be training 3-4 days per week, using the most effective strength and muscle building exercises, with easy to understand programming.

Each of the Main Compound Lifts (Squat, Bench Press, Deadlift, and Military Press) will be trained multiple times per week with varying intensities to allow for optimal recovery, while still getting in a lot of muscle-building work.

So, whether you choose too pack on the pounds or maintain the same bodyweight, these workouts will force you to get stronger like never before through proper training and recovery!

Plus, you will constantly progress at your own pace until you are repping out your old maxes!

No matter your previous experience, this strength training program will absolutely push you to the next level!

No need for tricks or special supplements. Just smart programming and hard work!

All you have to do is take on the challenge and put in the work!

# PROGRAM DETAILS

**This program is based on the Mathias Method Strength System.**

In the Mathias Method Strength System we don't train muscle groups. We train movements and base our workouts on improving one lift. This is because lifts like the squat, bench press, deadlift and military press are all full body lifts. They take your entire body working in unison to perfect and do not target one specific area.

By building up these powerful compound movements we will develop strength and muscle throughout our entire body.

We also believe in using only the most effective accessory exercises. Big bang exercises that build big muscle and big strength. Yeah, they are hard ones and they make you brutally strong too.

This training style may be different than what you are used to, but it is what has worked for me and countless others with the same goal of getting brutally strong.

The details of your training are discussed below.

## THE WARM-UP

Warm-ups are just what you think. They are simply meant too, warm-up your body for the intense work ahead, but not overly fatigue you.

If you are not used to doing some warm-up exercises before your main work, then it will be fatiguing at first until your body gets more conditioned. This is part of developing the work capacity to lift heavy weight, so do not skip this just because you do not feel like it. If you want to get stronger, you're gonna have to put in the work no matter how you "feel".

Warm-ups should be relatively easy and never done to failure.

Every workout you do should start with 1-3 rounds of *The Daily 30* (see page 4) to practice your movement patterns and improve mobility while you warm-up. This may seem unnecessary, but it will do wonders for your strength and help to alleviate any muscle or joint pain you have.

Get my *How To Warm-Up Properly for Strength Training Guide* (see page 4) for best results!

## Technique Work

Exercise Technique is a crucial part of any movement based training program. Without proper technique your body will learn improper movement patterns that can hold back your strength and cause injury.

Technique is so important that it should be checked and improved every time you start a training session!

Your technique work is still part of your warm-up and therefore only light weights (<50% of your maximum) should be used to prevent over fatiguing yourself. The focus is on improving your movement pattern by utilizing perfect form, under controlled movements.

The main goals of this exercise is to prepare your body for the more intense work ahead, build up weaknesses and increase work capacity.

You should do only 3 sets of 5 perfect reps. Again, the goals are to improve the motion of this exercise and better prepare your body for the work ahead, not to pre-fatigue those muscles.

After completing your Technique Work, you are ready to begin your workout!

Start with your first exercise by doing the same number of repetitions you plan to train with for that day. If you are doing 5 reps for your working sets, do all your warm-ups with 5 reps. Start with a low intensity and work your way up slowly.

## Main Lifts

The main lift, or main lifts, of any given workout is the focus point of the session. This is where the most effort should be placed in order to better improve this movement. All of the training before and after these lifts is set to better improve the main exercise.

The main exercise should be a standard motion that improves performance in your chosen sport.

For your main lift, stick with doing 5x5, starting at a weight you can do 10 reps with or about 70% of your max. Use the same weight on all 5 sets. For the 5th set, you can do an AMRAP (As Many Reps As Possible…with good form), but always save 1 or 2 reps in the tank so that you never reach failure.

To continue progressing forward, both in strength and muscular development, you should constantly be doing more work than before. To do this, add 5-10 pounds to each of your main lifts (Squat, Bench Press, Deadlift, Military Press) every week until you can no longer do all 5 reps with good form, then decrease by 10-20 pounds the following session and start the progression again. Do this for 6 months to a year, then you can change things up.

The first few weeks will likely feel pretty easy, and that is the idea. Lift explosive and have perfect form that will then carry over into the heavier weeks. This will ensure you are always progressing and are given a break when needed to avoid any strength plateaus.

Remember to always keep good form.

## Main Accessory

Your main accessory is complimentary to your main lift. It is another main lift, related to the lift you just did, but done at a much lower intensity. The purpose of this movement is to give you more practice in doing your main lifts, and adding in work to help build them up without over fatiguing you before the next session.

When doing a main lift only once per week, there is not enough work for most people to progress. By adding in some more light work, you accumulate more work volume which adds up to more strength.

For this lift, it is very important that you keep it under 70% of your maximum. The goal of this lift is to add in work, not obliterate your muscles to where you can't recover enough to progress before your next session. Keep it light and work on your technique.

I recommend you use 50-70% of your maximum on this lift and only do 5 reps per set. Start with 50% and if it is too easy you can slowly work your way up in weight.

## Accessory Work

For accessory work, you can do any exercises that you feel help you get stronger. The exercises listed in this section are recommendations that work best for most people. Build strength with the main lifts, then train your weaknesses and do muscle building exercises for accessory stuff.

Accessory work is in place to improve the main lifts performed that day, improve muscle weaknesses and increase the volume of work performed.

Accessory work should be performed with low to moderate intensity to allow for optimal muscle growth and proper technique. It is important to always be in control of the weight during any exercise being performed.

For accessory lifts, choose a weight that keeps you within the given rep ranges. Stick with the same weight while trying to add reps over time. When you reach the top of the allotted rep range, increase the weight slightly (5-10 pounds) and again focus on increasing your reps. This will add up your total work over time and make for a smoother progression forward.

Always stop 1-2 repetitions before failure on all sets other than the last, which can be taken to near failure if desired.

You can vary the intensity and repetitions slightly, just don't go to failure for any particular muscle group more than once per week, if at all. Lifting to failure is a good muscle building tool, when done infrequently, but doing it too often teaches your muscle to fail, or give up. You also lose form as you start to fail, so use it infrequently, if at all.

## Cardio/Conditioning

Conditioning, or cardio, is not necessary for this program, but can assist with dropping weight and improving recovery, if needed. Just DO NOT do cardio to warm-up! Get my *How To Warm-Up Properly for Strength Training Guide* to learn how to warm-up properly.

Conditioning, is any form of work that improves your cardiovascular health and total work capacity while assisting with the goals of training. Some examples of conditioning are; jogging, sprints, jump rope, battle ropes, light circuit training, a daily WOD, sled dragging, or just manual labor.

Conditioning is meant to increase the ability for your body to withstand work and become stronger.

If you have low cardiovascular health and little muscular endurance then the amount of work your body can withstand is greatly diminished, along with your ability to become stronger. So, if you have a low work capacity, you should add in conditioning work until it improves.

Conditioning can be performed 2-4 times per week for 10-20 minutes at a time. You may utilize high intensity interval training (HIIT) or moderate intensity steady state training.

With high intensity intervals, work to rest should be at a 1:1 or 1:2 ratio. For moderate intensity steady state conditioning, the body should stay in motion throughout the entire time with little to no resistance in order to sustain a raised heart rate during the time used.

It is best to do conditioning immediately after all accessory work, just before mobility work. This will add to the work already done in the workout and allow for the greatest increase in muscular advancement.

Conditioning can also be done on non-training days if preferred, but should then be done for 20-30 minutes.

Remember, conditioning is meant to condition your body, not break it down beyond what your body can repair before the next training session. Use relatively light loads and just keep moving.

## Mobility Work

A healthy joint and muscle must be strong and flexible. If there is too much strength without flexibility then there is a higher potential for ligament, muscle and joint tears. If there is too much flexibility without enough strength, then the joint is unstable and has a higher potential for dislocation. Therefore, to maintain a high level of performance there must be strength and flexibility throughout the body.

For Mobility Work in this program, do 10+ minutes of stretching at the end of every workout used increase flexibility, prevent injury and improve recovery. Focus on stretching out the muscle you just worked, or other tight areas.

It can be as simple as doing just 2-3 stretches for 2 minutes each to fix your elbow, shoulder, ankle, or hip pain.

Mobility work can also be replaced by yoga or any other activity that improves your body's ability to move as intended without pain, such as foam rolling.

It is best to mobilize right after a workout, but it can also be done on non-training days.

The goal is to get at least 30-40 minutes of mobilization done weekly to enhance your recovery and performance. That is just 10 minutes 3-4 times per week.

Go to [MathiasMethod.com](MathiasMethod.com) to learn how to do the best and most effective mobility exercises for athletes and lifters.

# Weekly Training Schedule

This Base Of Strength Training Program is designed for you to workout 4 days per week. Here is the training split I have found to be most effective for this program.

**Day 1 - Workout 1:** Squat Training

**Day 2 - Workout 2:** Bench Press Training

**Day 3 -** Rest & Recover

**Day 4 - Workout 3:** Deadlift Training

**Day 5 - Workout 4:** Military Press Training

**Day 6 -** Rest & Recover

**Day 7 -** Rest & Recover

*This weekly schedule can vary as needed, but is best in this form.

**Try to have at least 1 rest day after 1-2 training days in a row.

If you can only workout 3 days per week you can drop workout 4 and just rotate the other 3 workouts to where you are doing Bench Press Training every other workout.

For example, one week you will do Workouts 1,2 and 3, then the next week you will do Workout 2, 1, and 2 again.

## Don't forget to train with a partner!

Training with a partner(s) is always better. So, try to include someone else in your training to help keep you accountable and push you to become better.

Whether they have more experience than you or less, it is always better to have someone else to get stronger with.

If you need too, you can even find a partner at the gym and make a new friend! We are all stronger together!

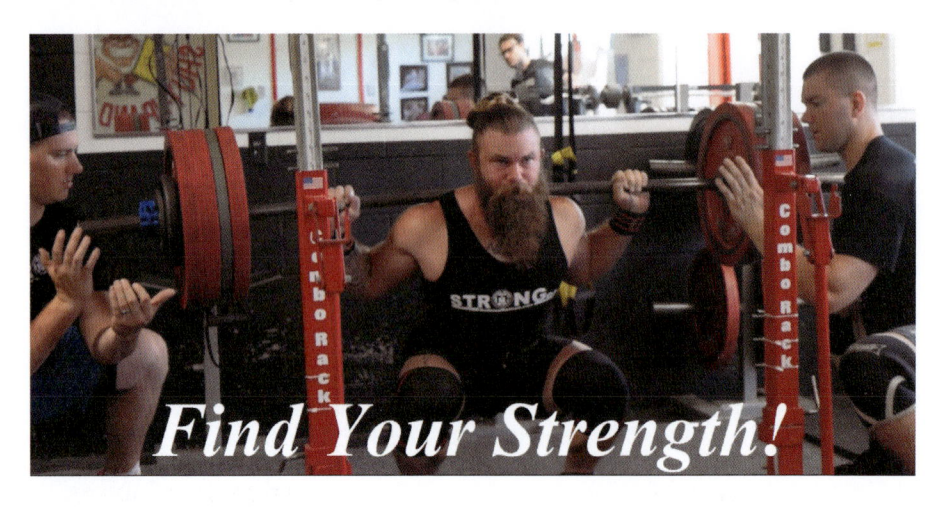

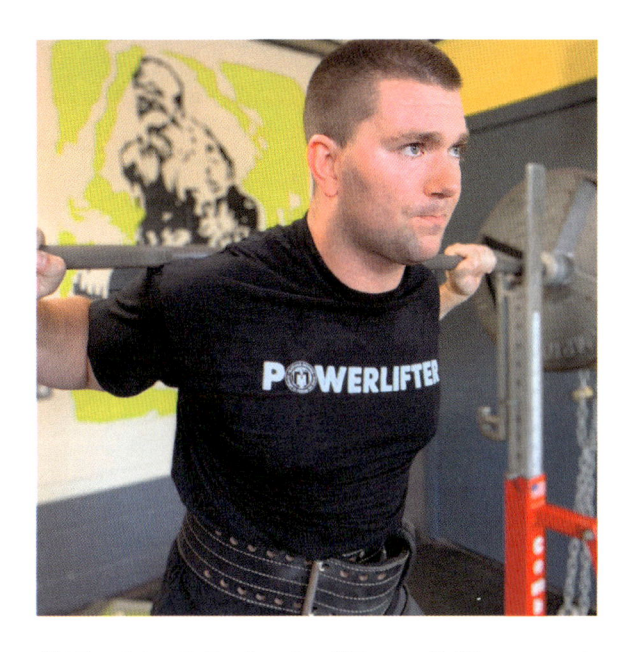

#MathiasMethod   #BaseOfStrength

**Follow @MathiasMethod on Social Media
and tag us in your #BaseOfStrength workout clips!**

**Also, feel free to reach out anytime with your questions
or technique checks!**

# Workouts

# Workout 1 - Squat Training

**Technique Work (<50%):**

Pause Squat                     3 x 5

**Main Lift (>70%):**

Squat                           5 x 5

**Main Accessory (<70%):**

Deadlift                        4 x 5

**Accessory Work:**

Leg Press                       4 x 10-15
Barbell Rows                    4 x 8-10
Dumbbell Curls                  4 x 10-15
Planks                          3 x 60 sec.

Cardio/Conditioning             10-20 min.

Mobility Work                   10+ min.


Go to [MathiasMethod.com](MathiasMethod.com) for in-depth exercise how to's.

# Workout 2 - Bench Press Training

**Technique Work (<50%):**

| | |
|---|---|
| Pause Bench Press | 3 x 5 |

**Main Lift (>70%):**

| | |
|---|---|
| Bench Press | 5 x 5 |

**Main Accessory (<70%):**

| | |
|---|---|
| Military Press | 4 x 5 |

**Accessory Work:**

| | |
|---|---|
| Dumbbell Press | 4 x 8-10 |
| Triceps Press Downs | 4 x 10-15 |
| Face Pulls | 4 x 10-15 |
| | |
| Cardio/Conditioning | 10-20 min. |
| | |
| Mobility Work | 10+ min. |

Go to [MathiasMethod.com](MathiasMethod.com) for in-depth exercise how to's.

# Workout 3 - Deadlift Training

**Technique Work (<50%):**

Deadlift                                3 x 5

**Main Lift (>70%):**

Deadlift                                5 x 5

**Main Accessory (<70%):**

Squat                                   4 x 5

**Accessory Work:**

Dumbbell Rows                           4 x 8-10
Lat Pull-Downs                          4 x 10-15
Hammer Curls                            3 x 8-10
Side Planks                             3 x 30 sec. each side

Cardio/Conditioning                     10-20 min.

Mobility Work                           10+ min.


Go to MathiasMethod.com for in-depth exercise how to's.

# Workout 4 - Military Press Training

**Technique Work (<50%):**

Military Press  3 x 5

**Main Lift (>70%):**

Military Press  5 x 5

**Main Accessory (<70%):**

Bench Press  4 x 5

**Accessory Work:**

Triceps Skull Crushers  4 x 10-15
Dumbbell Reverse Flyes  4 x 10-15
Dumbbell Lateral Raises  4 x 10-15

Cardio/Conditioning  10-20 min.

Mobility Work  10+ min.

Go to [MathiasMethod.com](MathiasMethod.com) for in-depth exercise how to's.

# Program FAQ's

## How Long Should I Rest Between Sets?

Different rest periods are used for different purposes. Depending on your goals rest periods will vary. Less rest is typically used with lighter loads and promotes greater conditioning. Longer rest periods are typically used with heavier loads to allow for more recovery and promote strength.

It takes about 3-5 minutes for your Phosphagen system to be prepared for another fatiguing strength set, but do not waste your whole training session waiting around too long. For most lifts just begin again when you are ready, within reason. The only rest needed between exercises is the time it takes to set up.

This program focuses on strength so rest periods should be as long as needed for your 5x5 main lifts (Generally 2-3 minutes, but can be up to 5 minutes).

For accessory work, rest periods should be between 1-2 minutes.

- **Main Lifts (5x5)** = As long as needed up to 5 Minutes
- **Accessory Work** = 1-2 minutes

## Can I Use Equipment?

Equipment in training is anything that assists you in lifting heavier loads. This could be very light assistant gear that has little to no impact on increasing loads, such as sleeves, all the way up to extremely supportive gear, such as lifting suits. One of the most common pieces of equipment to be used is a lifting belt. When used properly, a lifting belt allows you to better brace your core for stabilization by increasing the intra-abdominal pressure placed on your spine. By increasing stabilization you are enabled to lift heavier loads. Equipment in this form is very useful but can also have adverse effects when used improperly.

If any one piece of equipment is used too frequently, then it will limit your body's ability to grow stronger in that area. Essentially, the equipment will become a crutch that then must be used every time training occurs in order to keep up with the strength developed in other areas. The most effective way to use equipment is only when it is necessary. For example, when using light to moderate loads, or during your warm-up, avoid using any equipment at all to bring up strength in all areas. Then when you put on equipment for maximal loads you will be that much stronger.

Even if you have an injury, only use the equipment when you need it. If your injury does not hurt, then do not cover it up with equipment. Allow it to grow stronger, within reason. When you are building strength, use little to no equipment. When you are testing strength, use whatever you can to improve your lift.

## Why Can't I Push Myself Until Failure?

There are two forms of failure in strength training; technical and absolute. Technical failure is the point in which you can no longer perform a repetition with reasonably perfect technique. This commonly occurs 1-2 repetitions before absolute failure. Absolute failure is when no more repetitions can be completed without assistance.

Failure, in both forms, should not occur too often. It is good to know what failure feels like when lifting so you know you are training hard, but most of the repetitions performed should be done with reasonably perfect technique to build the most amount of strength.

For any given exercise, technical failure should only be reached on the last 1-2 sets if at all. This allows for maximal stimuli of the muscle fibers and central nervous system while still performing safe technique. It is relatively safe to reach technical failure without much chance of injury and the muscles will likely be able to recover before your next training session.

Reaching absolute failure too often will result in a much greater chance for injury and a much longer recovery period that may extend beyond the next training session. Absolute failure should only be reached once per month, if at all, to get the most benefit from your training. The idea for strength training is too accumulate volume for growth over multiple training sessions per week utilizing perfect practice. Reaching failure can slow progress and cause a plateau.

At least 85-90% of training repetitions for any given exercise should be performed with reasonably perfect technique. 10-15% can be utilized for failure, with less than 5% being absolute failure. This will ensure safety while gaining the most amount of strength over time.

**If you have any more questions, you can email me anytime at:**
ryan@mathiasmethod.com

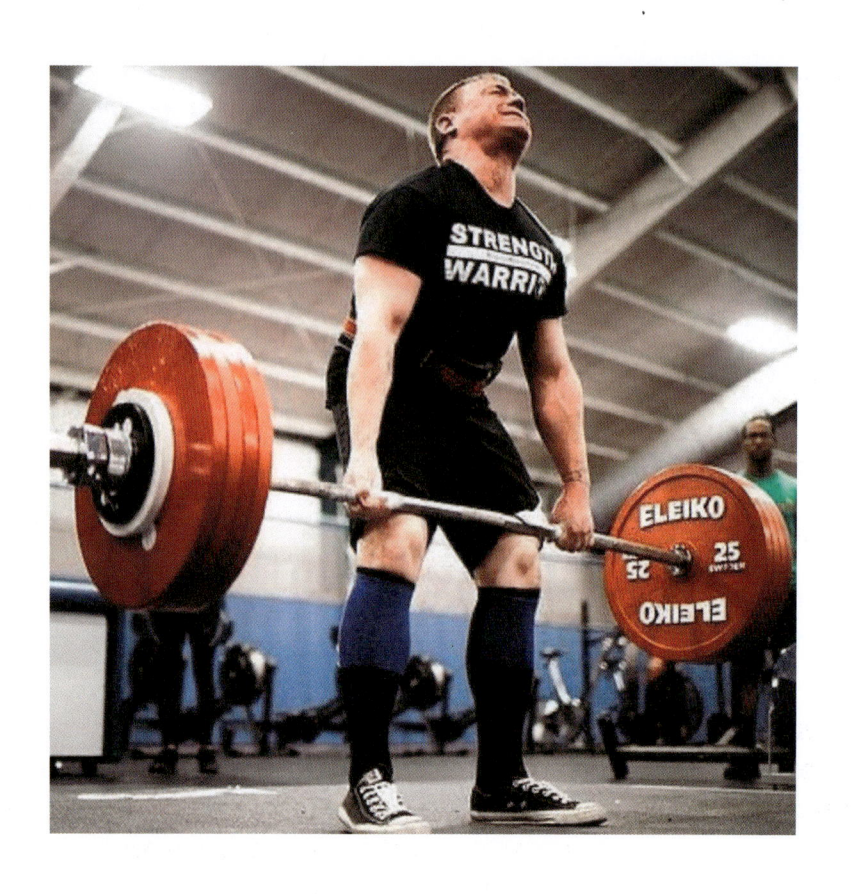

# Final Note

No matter where you are along your Strength Journey, whether you just started or are an experienced Strength Warrior, always remember the importance of strength. Be humble enough to slow down when needed, and take a step back to regain what you may have lost.

Strength will always lead you forward and never hold you back. Our strength is what makes us who we are, in and out of the gym. Build your strength, and never let it go.

## WOULD YOU DO ME A FAVOR?

**Thank you for reading and I hope you learned a lot!**

Before you go, please do me a HUGE favor and take a moment to let me know what you liked most about this book by leaving a review on Amazon! I read all my reviews and I love hearing how my work has helped others.

Plus, it helps more people learn what they can get from this book!

If you were not completely satisfied with the content of this book please let me know by emailing me directly and I will be happy to answer your questions or help you further.

Thank you, and keep getting stronger my friends!

# Email: ryan@mathiasmethod.com

Do you know someone that would benefit from this book?

**Please tell them about it!**

Everyone can benefit from getting stronger!

# More Books By Ryan J. Mathias

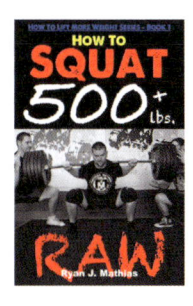

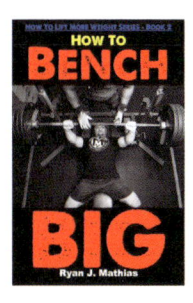

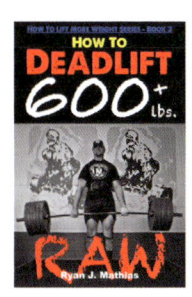

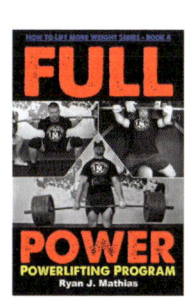

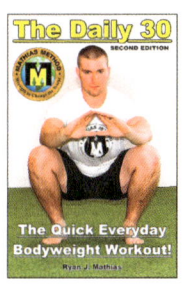

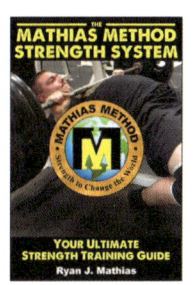

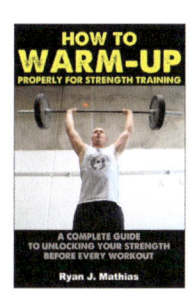

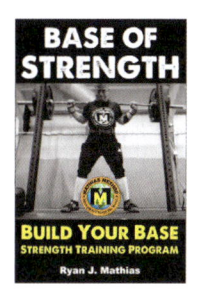

## Available on
## Amazon.com
### and
## StrengthWorld.store

## Follow The Strength Blog

We have over 200+ articles on how to get stronger and workout properly, in and out of the gym!

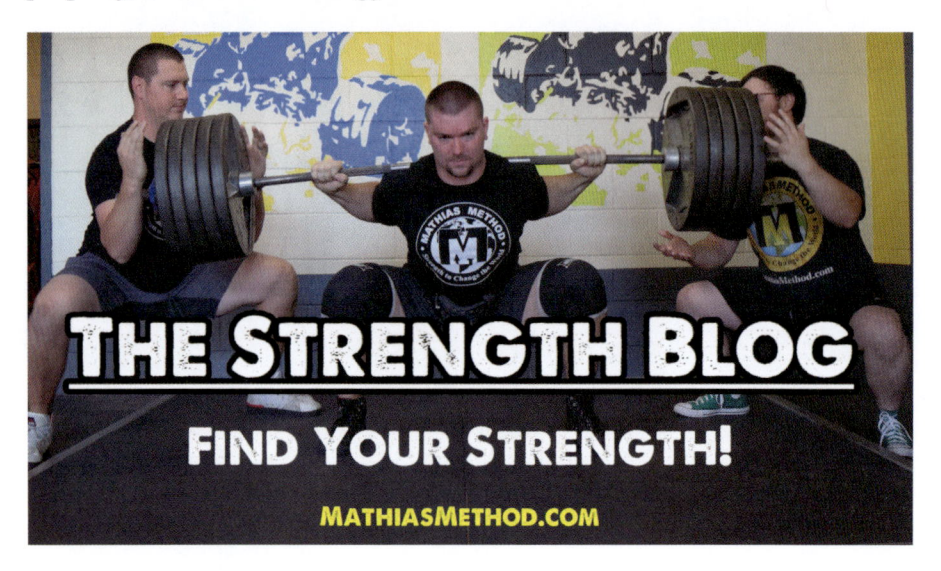

Go to MathiasMethod.com to follow the Strength Blog and get all the awesome NEW Content we put out!

- **New Articles**
- **Workout Programs**
- **Valuable Strength Training Resources!**

## FOLLOW US ON SOCIAL MEDIA

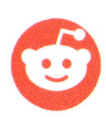

**Facebook:** @MathiasMethodStrength

**Instagram:** @MathiasMethod

**Twitter:** @MathiasMethod

**YouTube:** @MathiasMethodStrength

**Reddit:** u/mathiasmethod

## Thank You

Thank you to all those that read this information and use it to help others. My mission is to help as many people as I can change the world through strength and I know I can't do it alone. So, thank you for standing with me.

## Special Thank You to

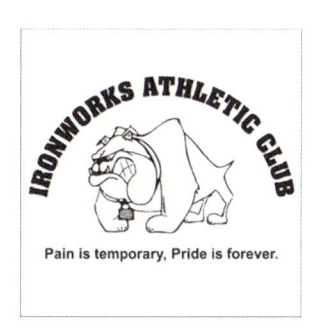

### Ironworks Gym

153 South Auburn St.
Grass Valley, CA 95945

PHONE #: (530) 272-9462

**Home of the Mathias Method Strength Warriors!**

Thank you for allowing us to use your awesome facility to help make the world a stronger place!

# Check out our Strength Apparel at
## StrengthWorld.store

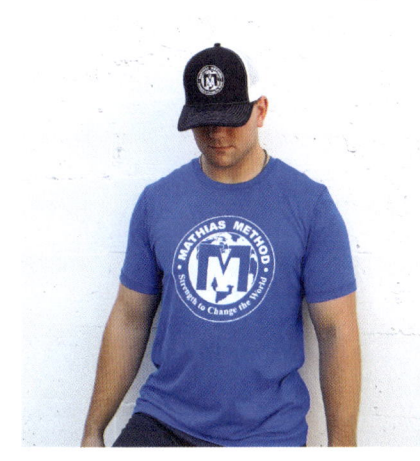

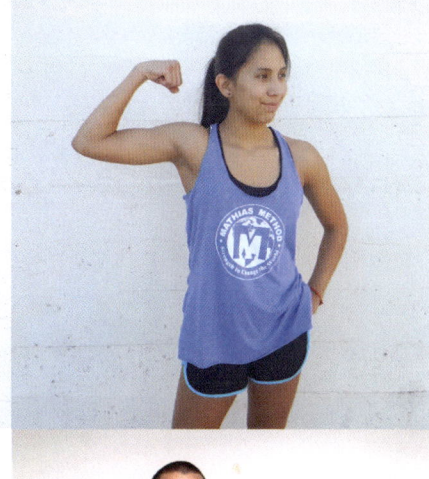

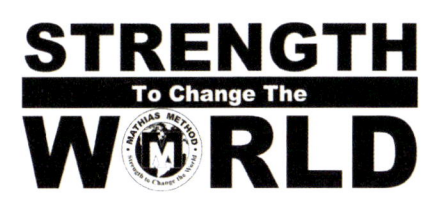

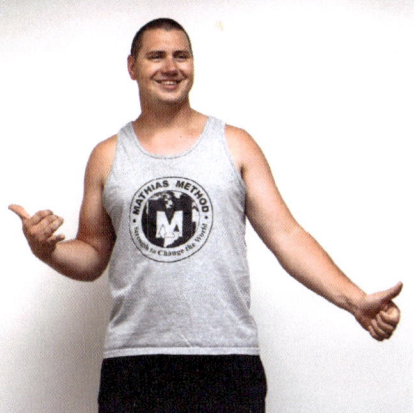

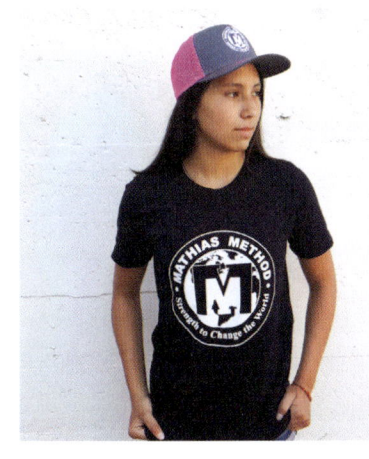

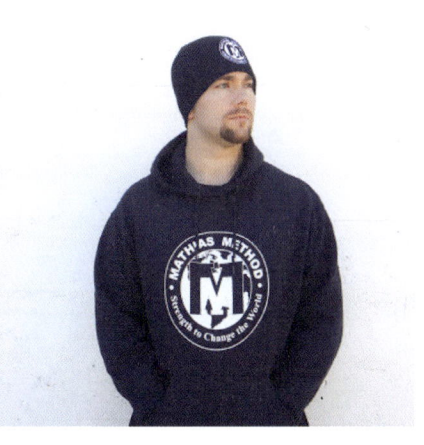

Use Code "BaseOfStrength10" for 10% OFF your first order as a gift for reading this book!

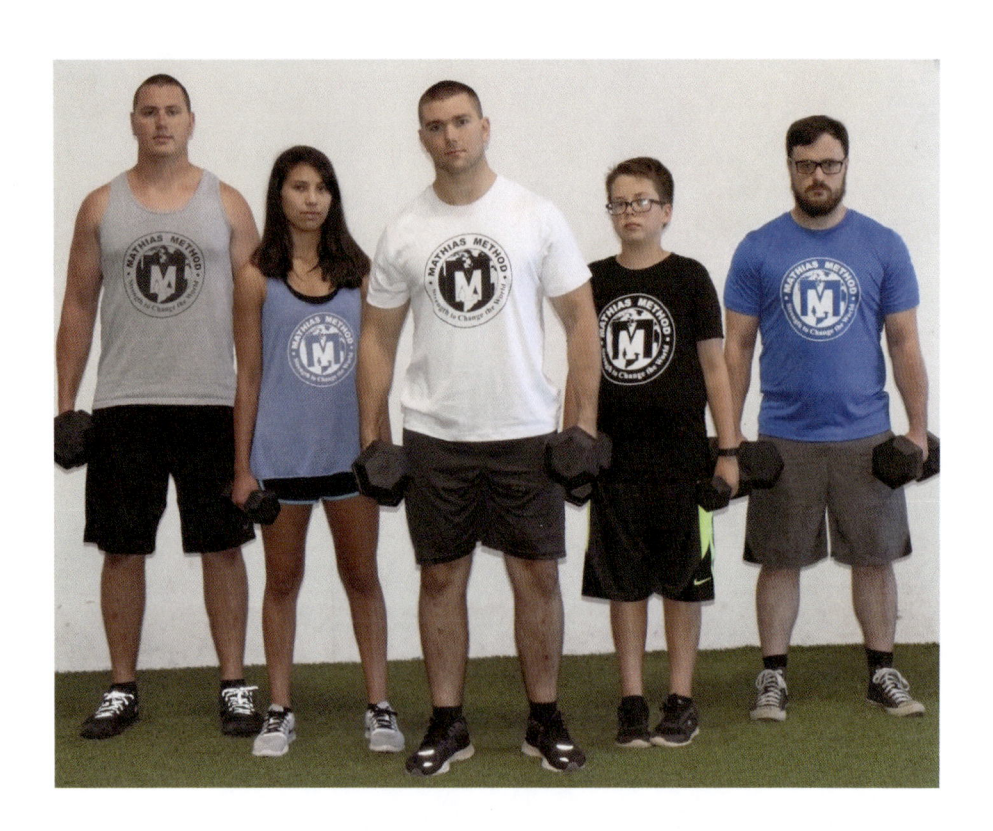

# Stand Strong and Change Your World!

© 2021 Mathias Method – All Rights Reserved.

Printed in Great Britain
by Amazon